COLOSTOMY

THINGS YOU SHOULD KNOW
(QUESTIONS AND ANSWERS)

By Rumi Michael Leigh

I0504408

Introduction

I would like to thank and congratulate you for purchasing this book, " *Colostomy, things you should know (questions and answers)*" series.

This book will help you understand, revise and have a good general knowledge and keywords in Colostomy.

Thanks again for purchasing this book, I hope you enjoy it!

Chapter 1

1) What is colostomy ?

- Colostomy is a surgical opening of the large intestine.

2) What are some of the reasons for a patient to have colostomy ?

- Some of the reasons for a patient to have colostomy are diverticulosis, Crohn's disease, colon cancer, rectal cancer, etc.

3) When does a colostomy become indispensable ?

- A colostomy becomes indispensable when a person can no longer evacuate feces in a natural way.

4) How many types of colostomy are there ?

- There are two types of colostomy.

5) What are the types of colostomy ?

- The types of colostomy are transverse colostomy and sigmoidostomy.

6) Is colostomy definitive ?

- No, colostomy is not always definitive, it could also be temporary.

7) What is a temporary sigmoidostomy ?

- A temporary sigmoidostomy is when there is the preservation of part of the rectum and anus while waiting for healing.

8) What is a permanent sigmoidostomy ?

- A permanent sigmoidostomy is the removal of the rectum and anus.

9) What are the risks of colostomy ?

- Some risks of colostomy include bleeding, infection, prolapse, hernia, etc.

10) Does the intestine changes its functional mode after a colostomy ?

- No, the intestine functions as it does before a colostomy.

Chapter 2

1) What is the length of the large intestine ?

- The length of the large intestine is about 1.5 meters to 1.8 meters.

2) What is another name for the small bowel ?

- The small bowel is also called the small intestine.

3) What is the main function of the small intestine ?

- The main function of the small intestine is to absorb nutrients.

4) What is the length of the small intestine ?

- The length of the small intestine is about 6 to 7 meters long, but this could vary.

5) What are the main parts of the small intestine ?

- The main parts of the small intestine are the ileum, the jejunum and the duodenum.

6) What is another name for the large bowel ?

- The large bowel is also called the colon.

7) What are the main functions of the colon ?

- The colon absorbs water and eliminates food waste as feces.

8) What are the main parts of the large intestine ?

- The main parts of the large intestine are the cecum, the ascending colon, the transverse colon, the descending colon, the sigmoid, and the rectum.

9) What is the form of feces in the ascending colon?

- Feces is in a liquid form in the ascending colon.

10) What is the form of feces in the transverse colon?

- Feces is in a semi-liquid form in the transverse colon.

11) What is the form of feces in the descending colon?

- Feces is in a solid form in the descending colon.

Chapter 3

1) Is colostomy the same as ileostomy ?

- No, colostomy is not the same as ileostomy.

2) What part of the digestive tract is colostomy ?

- Colostomy is in the large intestine.

3) What part of the digestive tract is ileostomy ?

- Ileostomy is in the small intestine.

4) How is the stool in colostomy ?

- In colostomy, the stool is often pasty.

5) How is the stool in ileostomy ?

- In ileostomy, the stool is liquid.

6) Which has more gas emission, colostomy or ileostomy ?

- Colostomy has more gas emission. There is very little or no gas in ileostomy.

7) Are there various locations of colostomy ?

- Yes, there are various locations of colostomy.

8) What are the various locations of colostomy ?

- The various locations of colostomy are the ascending, descending, and sigmoid colon.

9) What part of the abdomen is the ascending colostomy located ?

- The ascending colostomy is located at the right area of the abdomen.

10) What part of the abdomen is the transverse colostomy located ?

- The transverse colostomy is located at the mid-abdominal area of the abdomen.

Chapter 4

1) What part of the abdomen is the descending colostomy located ?

- The descending colostomy is located at the upper left area of the abdomen.

2) What part of the abdomen is the sigmoid colostomy located ?

- The sigmoid colostomy is located at the lower left area of the abdomen.

3) How many types of transverse colostomies are there ?

- There are two types of transverse colostomies.

4) What are the two types of transverse colostomies?

- The two types of transverse colostomies are the loop transverse colostomy and the double-barrel transverse colostomy.

5) What is a double-barrel transverse colostomy ?

- A double-barrel transverse colostomy is the creation of two stomas.

6) What is a loop colostomy ?

- A loop colostomy is a temporary colostomy.

7) What kind of bags are used after a transverse colostomy ?

- Drainable bags are used after a transverse colostomy.

8) Can the irrigation method be used after a transverse colostomy ?

- No, the irrigation method cannot be used after a transverse colostomy.

9) The cecum is prolonged by ?

- The cecum is prolonged by the vermiform appendage.

10) Where is sigmoidostomy normally done ?

- Sigmoidostomy is normally done on the left side, on the lower side of the stomach.

11) What kind of bags are used after a sigmoidostomy ?

- After a sigmoidostomy, closed bags are used.

Chapter 5

1) What is a stoma ?

- A stoma is a surgical opening of a part of the body to allow evacuation.

2) Why is the location of the stoma done while the patient is in different positions such as laying down, sitting and standing before the operation procedure ?

- The location of the stoma is done while the patient is in different positions in order to facilitate care and to be sure that the stoma is away from the skin folds.

3) Can a person with stoma practice swimming ?

- Yes, a person with stoma can practice swimming but with precautions.

4) Is pregnancy possible with a stoma ?

- Yes, pregnancy is possible with a stoma.

5) Can a stoma cause vaginal retraction ?

- Yes, a stoma can cause the vagina to retract.

6) Can men have erection problems due to a stoma?

- Yes, men can have erection problems due to a stoma.

7) Can men have ejaculation problems due to a stoma ?

- Yes, men can have ejaculation problems due to a stoma.

8) Is a stoma painful ?

- No, a stoma is normally not painful.

9) Why is a stoma not painful ?

- A stoma is not painful because there are no nerve endings.

10) Can the passage of feces from the stoma be controlled ?

- No, the passage of feces from the stoma cannot be controlled.

Chapter 6

1) How many types of stoma are there ?

- There are 3 types of stoma.

2) What are the types of stoma ?

- The three types of stoma are colostomy, urostomy and ileostomy.

3) What is the function of the proximal stoma ?

- The function of the proximal stoma is to drain feces.

4) What is the function of the distal stoma ?

- The distal stoma is nonfunctional.

5) Is the proximal stoma functional ?

- Yes, the proximal stoma is functional.

6) What does the distal stoma drain ?

- The distal stoma drains mucus.

7) What should be the appearance of a stoma ?

- A stoma should be reddish, pinkish, and moist.

8) What is an abnormal appearance of a stoma ?

- An abnormal appearance of a stoma is a dark red color.

9) What does a dark red color signify in a stoma ?

- A dark red color signifies that there is deficiency of blood circulation in the stoma.

10) Is it normal for a stoma to be large after an operation ?

- Yes, it is normal for a stoma to be large after an operation, but it will decrease to a normal size after some weeks.

Chapter 7

1) What should be observed in a colostomy bag ?

- In a colostomy bag, the color, blood, odor, and the shape of the stool have to be observed.

2) What can be used to retain odors when evacuating intestinal gases ?

- To retain odors when evacuating intestinal gases, a carbon filter can be used.

3) Does an airtight pouch emit odors ?

- No, an airtight pouch does not emit odors.

4) What is the function of the skin barrier of a pouch?

- The skin barrier of a pouch protects the skin from contact with feces.

5) How can odors be reduced in a stoma bag ?

- Special tablets or liquids can be put in a stoma bag to reduce odors.

6) How often should a closed bag be changed ?

- It depends, a closed bag should be changed once, twice or more times a day.

7) Why should products containing alcohol not be used during a care treatment ?

- Alcohol-containing products should not be used during a care treatment as this can irritate the skin.

8) Who is an Ostomy nurse ?

- An Ostomy nurse is a specialized nurse that treats and educates patients about their stoma.

9) Why is unscented soap used in ostomy care ?

- Unscented soap is used in ostomy care in order to avoid skin irritation.

10) What water temperature should be used for ostomy care ?

- Warm water should be used for ostomy care.

Chapter 8

1) What is mycosis ?

- Mycosis is a fungal infection.

2) What is prolapse ?

- Prolapse is when an organ falls down from its original place.

3) What is hernia ?

- Hernia is the protrusion of an organ or a tissue through an abnormal opening.

4) What is colonic irrigation ?

- Colonic irrigation is the enema of the large intestine.

5) What causes flatulence ?

- The causes of flatulence are smoking, lactose intolerance, chewing gum, soft drinks, lack of physical activity, etc.

6) Name two types of anesthesia.

- A local and a general anesthesia.

7) What is a local anesthesia ?

- A local anesthesia is an anesthesia in a region of the body. The patient feels no pain at that region and the patient is awake.

8) What is a general anesthesia ?

- A general anesthesia is an anesthesia where the patient is not awake, does not feel any pain and is unconscious.

9) What is Crohn's disease ?

- Crohn's disease is a chronic inflammation of the digestive tract.

10) What are the signs and symptoms of Crohn's disease ?

- The signs and symptoms of Crohn's disease are fatigue, fever, skin inflammation, diarrhea, blood in stool, etc.

Chapter 9

1) What is Hirschsprung's disease ?

- Hirschsprung's disease is a disease that causes difficulty in passing stool.

2) What are the signs and symptoms of Hirschsprung's disease ?

- The signs and symptoms of Hirschsprung's disease are fatigue, diarrhea, swollen belly, constipation, vomiting, etc.

3) Who is likely to have Hirschsprung's disease ?

- Babies and young children are likely to have Hirschsprung's disease.

4) What is enterocolitis ?

- Enterocolitis is the inflammation of the small intestine and the large intestine.

5) What are the signs and symptoms of enterocolitis?

- The signs and symptoms of enterocolitis are a swollen abdomen, vomiting, blood in stool, etc.

6) Is colostomy done under local or general anesthesia?

- Colostomy is done under general anesthesia.

7) What is laparoscopy ?

-   Laparoscopy is a mini invasive surgical procedure done with a camera.

8) Name the two types of pouching system.

-   There is the one-piece pouching system and a two-piece pouching system.

9) What is the one-piece pouching system ?

-   The one-piece pouching system has a skin barrier that is attached to the pouch.

10) What is the two-piece pouching system ?

-   In the two-piece pouching system, the skin barrier is separate from the pouch.

Chapter 10

1) Why should the hair around the stoma be shaved?

- The hair around the stoma should be shaved because it helps the skin barrier of the pouch to stick properly.

2) Why should the skin around the stoma be dry after cleaning ?

- The skin around the stoma should be dry after cleaning in order to enable the pouching system to stick properly.

3) What is the use of the barrier ring in an ostomy bag pouch ?

- The barrier ring in an ostomy bag pouch protects the stoma.

4) What is a good rule to change the pouch ?

- A good rule to change the pouch is when it is a third full.

5) When should a patient with colostomy contact their doctor or ostomy nurse (sign of emergency)?

- A patient with colostomy should contact his/her doctor or ostomy nurse if he/she has signs such as inflammation, mycosis, hernia, allergy, absence of stool, retraction, stomach aches, bleeding and prolapses.

6) Can people with colostomy work ?

- Yes, a working life with colostomy is possible.

7) What kind of work should precautions be taken for a person with colostomy ?

- A person with colostomy should avoid lifting heavy objects (heavy weights).

8) What kind of sport should mostly be avoided for a person with colostomy ?

- Contact sports such as combat sports, etc. should be avoided for a person with colostomy.

9) Is a normal sex life possible after colostomy ?

- Yes, a normal sex life is possible after colostomy.

Conclusion

Thank you again for purchasing this book. I hope it has helped you in your journey to understanding Colostomy and how it affects the people around you who suffer from it.

Thank you.